THE TWELVE HEALERS

And Other Remedies

by

Edward Bach
M.B., B.S., M.R.C.S., L.R.C.P., D.P.H.

Copyright © 2017 Read Books Ltd.
This book is copyright and may not be
reproduced or copied in any way without
the express permission of the publisher in writing

British Library Cataloguing-in-Publication Data
A catalogue record for this book is available from the
British Library

INTRODUCTION

This system of treatment is the most perfect which has been given to mankind within living memory. It has the power to cure disease; and, in its simplicity, it may be used in the household.

It is its simplicity, combined with its all-healing effects, that is so wonderful.

No science, no knowledge is necessary, apart from the simple methods described herein; and they who will obtain the greatest benefit from this God-sent Gift will be those who keep it pure as it is; free from science, free from theories, for everthing in Nature is simple.

This system of healing, which has been Divinely revealed unto us, shows that it is our fears, our cares, our anxieties and such like that open the path to the invasion of illness. Thus by treating our fears, our cares, our worries and so on, we not only free ourselves from our illness, but the Herbs given unto us by the Grace of the Creator of all, in addition take away our fears and worries, and leave us happier and better in ourselves.

As the Herbs heal our fears, our anxieties, our worries, our faults and our failings, it is these we must seek, and then the disease, no matter what it is, will leave us.

There is little more to say, for the understanding mind will know all this, and may there be sufficient of those with understanding minds, unhampered by the trend of science, to use these Gifts of God for the relief and the blessing of those around them.

Thus, behind all disease lie our fears, our anxieties, our greed, our likes and dislikes. Let us seek these out and heal them, and with the healing of them will go the disease from which we suffer.

From time immemorial it has been known that Providential Means has placed in Nature the prevention and cure of disease, by means of divinely enriched herbs and plants and trees. The remedies of Nature given in this book have proved that they are blest above others in their work of mercy; and that they have been given the power to heal all types of illness and suffering.

In treating cases with these remedies no notice is taken of the nature of the disease. The individual is treated, and as he becomes well the disease goes, having been cast off by the increase of health.

All know that the same disease may have different effects on different people; it is the effects that need treatment, because they guide to the real cause.

The mind being the most delicate and sensitive part of the body, shows the onset and the course of disease much more definitely than the body, so that the outlook of mind is chosen as the guide as to which remedy or remedies are necessary.

In illness there is a change of mood from that in

ordinary life, and those who are observant can notice this change often before, and sometimes long before, the disease appears, and by treatment can prevent the malady ever appearing. When illness has been present for some time, again the mood of the sufferer will guide to the correct remedy.

Take no notice of the disease, think only of the outlook on life of the one in distress.

Thirty-eight different states are simply described: and there should be no difficulty either for oneself, or for another, to find that state or a mixture of states which are present, and so to be able to give the required remedies to effect a cure.

The title, *The Twelve Healers*, has been retained for this book, as it is familiar to many readers.

The relief of suffering was so certain and beneficial, even when there were only twelve remedies, that it was deemed necessary to bring these before the attention of the public at the time, without waiting for the discovery of the remaining twenty-six, which complete the series. The original twelve are indicated by asterisks.

THE REMEDIES
And the reasons given for each

THE 38 REMEDIES

are placed under the following

7 HEADINGS

		Page
1.	For Fear	9
2.	For Uncertainty	11
3.	For Insufficient Interest in Present Circumstances	13
4.	For Loneliness	16
5.	For Those Over-sensitive to Influences and Ideas	17
6.	For Despondency or Despair	19
7.	For Over-Care for Welfare of Others	22

FOR THOSE WHO HAVE FEAR

*ROCK ROSE

The remedy of emergency for cases where there even appears no hope. In accident or sudden illness, or when the patient is very frightened or terrified, or if the condition is serious enough to cause great fear to those around. If the patient is not conscious the lips may be moistened with the remedy. Other remedies in addition may also be required, as, for example, if there is unconsciousness, which is a deep, sleepy state, Clematis; if there is torture, Agrimony, and so on.

*MIMULUS

Fear of wordly things, illness, pain, accidents, poverty, of dark, of being alone, of misfortune. The fears of everyday life. These people quietly and secretly bear their dread, they do not freely speak of it to others.

CHERRY PLUM

Fear of the mind being over-strained, of reason giving way, of doing fearful and dreaded things, not wished and known wrong, yet there comes the thought and impulse to do them.

ASPEN

Vague unknown fears, for which there can be given no explanation, no reason.

Yet the patient may be terrified of something terrible going to happen, he knows not what.

These vague unexplainable fears may haunt by night or day.

Sufferers are often afraid to tell their trouble to others.

RED CHESTNUT

For those who find it difficult not to be anxious for other people.

Often they have ceased to worry about themselves, but for those of whom they are fond they may suffer much, frequently anticipating that some unfortunate thing may happen to them.

FOR THOSE WHO SUFFER UNCERTAINTY

*CERATO

Those who have not sufficient confidence in themselves to make their own decisions.

They constantly seek advice from others, and are often misguided.

*SCLERANTHUS

Those who suffer much from being unable to decide between two things, first one seeming right then the other.

They are usually quiet people, and bear their difficulty alone, as they are not inclined to discuss it with others.

*GENTIAN

Those who are easily discouraged. They may be progressing well in illness or in the affairs of their daily life, but any small delay or hindrance to progress causes doubt and soon disheartens them.

GORSE

Very great hopelessness, they have given up belief that more can be done for them.

Under persuasion or to please others they may try different treatments, at the same time assuring those around that there is so little hope of relief.

HORNBEAM

For those who feel that they have not sufficient strength, mentally or physically, to carry the burden of life placed upon them; the affairs of every day seem too much for them to accomplish, though they generally succeed in fulfilling their task.

For those who believe that some part, of mind or body, needs to be strengthened before they can easily fulfil their work.

WILD OAT

Those who have ambitions to do something of prominence in life, who wish to have much experience, and to enjoy all that which is possible for them, to take life to the full.

Their difficulty is to determine what occupation to follow; as although their ambitions are strong, they have no calling which appeals to them above all others.

This may cause delay and dissatisfaction.

NOT SUFFICIENT INTEREST IN PRESENT CIRCUMSTANCES

*CLEMATIS

Those who are dreamy, drowsy, not fully awake, no great interest in life. Quiet people, not really happy in their present circumstances, living more in the future than in the present; living in hopes of happier times, when their ideals may come true. In illness some make little or no effort to get well, and in certain cases may even look forward to death, in the hope of better times; or maybe, meeting again some beloved one whom they have lost.

HONEYSUCKLE

Those who live much in the past, perhaps a time of great happiness, or memories of a lost friend, or ambitions which have not come true. They do not expect further happiness such as they have had.

WILD ROSE

Those who without apparently sufficient reason become resigned to all that happens, and just glide through life, take it as it is, without any effort to improve things and find some joy. They have surrendered to the struggle of life without complaint.

OLIVE

Those who have suffered much mentally or physically and are so exhausted and weary that they feel they have no more strength to make any effort. Daily life is hard work for them, without pleasure.

WHITE CHESTNUT

For those who cannot prevent thoughts, ideas, arguments which they do not desire from entering their minds. Usually at such times when the interest of the moment is not strong enough to keep the mind full.

Thoughts which worry and will remain, or if for a time thrown out, will return. They seem to circle round and round and cause mental torture.

The presence of such unpleasant thoughts drives out peace and interferes with being able to think only of the work or pleasure of the day.

MUSTARD

Those who are liable to times of gloom, or even despair, as though a cold dark cloud overshadowed them and hid the light and the joy of life. It may not be possible to give any reason or explanation for such attacks.

Under these conditions it is almost impossible to appear happy or cheerful.

CHESTNUT BUD

For those who do not take full advantage of observation and experience, and who take a longer time than others to learn the lessons of daily life.

Whereas one experience would be enough for some, such people find it necessary to have more, sometimes several, before the lesson is learnt.

Therefore, to their regret, they find themselves having to make the same error on different occasions when once would have been enough, or observation of others could have spared them even that one fault.

LONELINESS

*WATER VIOLET

For those who in health or illness like to be alone. Very quiet people, who move about without noise, speak little, and then gently. Very independent, capable and self-reliant. Almost free of the opinions of others. They are aloof, leave people alone and go their own way. Often clever and talented. Their peace and calmness is a blessing to those around them.

*IMPATIENS

Those who are quick in thought and action and who wish all things to be done without hesitation or delay. When ill they are anxious for a hasty recovery.

They find it very difficult to be patient with people who are slow, as they consider it wrong and a waste of time, and they will endeavour to make such people quicker in all ways.

They often prefer to work and think alone, so that they can do everything at their own speed.

HEATHER

Those who are always seeking the companionship of anyone who may be available, as they find it necessary to discuss their own affairs with others, no matter whom it may be. They are very unhappy if they have to be alone for any length of time.

OVER-SENSITIVE TO INFLUENCES AND IDEAS

*AGRIMONY

The jovial, cheerful, humorous people who love peace and are distressed by argument or quarrel, to avoid which they will agree to give up much.

Though generally they have troubles and are tormented and restless and worried in mind or in body, they hide their cares behind their humour and jesting and are considered very good friends to know. They often take alcohol or drugs in excess, to stimulate themselves and help themselves bear their trials with cheerfulness.

*CENTAURY

Kind, quiet, gentle people who are over-anxious to serve others. They overtax their strength in their endeavours.

Their wish so grows upon them that they become more servants than willing helpers. Their good nature leads them to do more than their own share of work, and in so doing they may neglect their own particular mission in life.

WALNUT

For those who have definite ideals and ambitions in life and are fulfilling them, but on rare occasions are tempted to be led away from their own ideas, aims and work by the enthusiasm, convictions or strong opinions of others.

The remedy gives constancy and protection from outside influences.

HOLLY

For those who are sometimes attacked by thoughts of such kind as jealousy, envy, revenge, suspicion.

For the different forms of vexation.

Within themselves they may suffer much, often when there is no real cause for their unhappiness.

FOR DESPONDENCY OR DESPAIR

LARCH

For those who do not consider themselves as good or capable as those around them, who expect failure, who feel that they will never be a success, and so do not venture or make a strong enough attempt to succeed.

PINE

For those who blame themselves. Even when successful they think they could have done better, and are never content with their efforts or the results. They are hard-working and suffer much from the faults they attach to themselves.

Sometimes if there is any mistake it is due to another, but they will claim responsibility even for that.

ELM

Those who are doing good work, are following the calling of their life and who hope to do something of importance, and this often for the benefit of humanity.

At times there may be periods of depression when

they feel that the task they have undertaken is too difficult, and not within the power of a human being.

SWEET CHESTNUT

For those moments which happen to some people when the anguish is so great as to seem to be unbearable.

When the mind or body feels as if it had borne to the uttermost limit of its endurance, and that now it must give way.

When it seems there is nothing but destruction and annihilation left to face.

STAR OF BETHLEHEM

For those in great distress under conditions which for a time produce great unhappiness.

The shock of serious news, the loss of someone dear, the fright following an accident, and such like.

For those who for a time refuse to be consoled, this remedy brings comfort.

WILLOW

For those who have suffered adversity or misfortune and find these difficult to accept, without complaint or resentment, as they judge life much by the success which it brings.

They feel that they have not deserved so great a trial, that it was unjust, and they become embittered.

They often take less interest and are less active in

those things of life which they had previously enjoyed.

OAK

For those who are struggling and fighting strongly to get well, or in connection with the affairs of their daily life. They will go on trying one thing after another, though their case may seem hopeless.

They will fight on. They are discontented with themselves if illness interferes with their duties or helping others.

They are brave people, fighting against great difficulties, without loss of hope or effort.

CRAB APPLE

This is the remedy of cleansing.

For those who feel as if they had something not quite clean about themselves.

Often it is something of apparently little importance: in others there may be more serious disease which is almost disregarded compared to the one thing on which they concentrate.

In both types they are anxious to be free from the one particular thing which is greatest in their minds and which seems so essential to them that it should be cured.

They become despondent if treatment fails.

Being a cleanser, this remedy purifies wounds if the patient has reason to believe that some poison has entered which must be drawn out.

OVER-CARE FOR WELFARE OF OTHERS

*CHICORY

Those who are very mindful of the needs of others they tend to be over-full of care for children, relatives, friends, always finding something that should be put right. They are continually correcting what they consider wrong, and enjoy doing so. They desire that those for whom they care should be near them.

*VERVAIN

Those with fixed principles and ideas, which they are confident are right, and which they very rarely change.

They have a great wish to convert all around them to their own views of life.

They are strong of will and have much courage when they are convinced of those things that they wish to teach.

In illness they struggle on long after many would have given up their duties.

VINE

Very capable people, certain of their own ability, confident of success.

Being so assured, they think that it would be for the benefit of others if they could be persuaded to do things as they themselves do, or as they are certain is right. Even in illness they will direct their attendants.

They may be of great value in emergency.

BEECH

For those who feel the need to see more good and beauty in all that surrounds them. And, although much appears to be wrong, to have the ability to see the good growing within. So as to be able to be more tolerant, lenient and understanding of the different way each individual and all things are working to their own final perfection.

ROCK WATER

Those who are very strict in their way of living; they deny themselves many of the joys and pleasures of life because they consider it might interfere with their work.

They are hard masters to themselves. They wish to be well and strong and active, and will do anything which they believe will keep them so. They hope to be examples which will appeal to others who may then follow their ideas and be better as a result.

For those who wish to treat themselves and others, or those who wish to pursue the subject further, the Bach Centre can provide general information and order sheets related to the individual or complete sets of stock remedies, coloured illustrations, books and the News Letter. Names and addresses of foreign distributors are also available.

Enquiries to:
Bach Flower Remedies®
Dr Edward Bach Centre
Mount Vernon
Wallingford
Oxon, OX10 0PZ
England

Where Dr Bach lived and worked and discovered his healing flowers in the surrounding fields and hedgerows.

(A S.A.E. would be appreciated from U.K. enquirers.)

The English and botanical name of each remedy is as follows:

AGRIMONY	*Agrimonia eupatoria*
ASPEN	*Populus tremula*
BEECH	*Fagus sylvatica*
CENTAURY	*Centaurium umbellatum*
CERATO	*Ceratostigma willmottiana*
CHERRY PLUM	*Prunus cerasifera*
CHESTNUT BUD	*AEsculus hippocastanum*
CHICORY	*Cichorium intybus*
CLEMATIS	*Clematis vitalba*
CRAB APPLE	*Malus pumila*
ELM	*Ulmus procera*
GENTIAN	*Gentiana amarella*
GORSE	*Ulex europoeus*
HEATHER	*Calluna vulgaris*
HOLLY	*Ilex aquifolium*
HONEYSUCKLE	*Lonicera caprifolium*
HORNBEAM	*Carpinus betulus*
IMPATIENS	*Impatiens glandulifera*
LARCH	*Larix decidua*
MIMULUS	*Mimulus guttatus*
MUSTARD	*Sinapis arvensis*
OAK	*Quercus robur*
OLIVE	*Olea europoea*
PINE	*Pinus sylvestris*
RED CHESTNUT	*AEsculus carnea*
ROCK ROSE	*Helianthemum nummularium*
ROCK WATER	*(see page 28)*

SCLERANTHUS	*Scleranthus annuus*
STAR OF BETHLEHEM	*Ornithogalum umbetelatum*
SWEET CHESTNUT	*Castanea sativa*
VERVAIN	*Verbena officinalis*
VINE	*Vitis vinifera*
WALNUT	*Juglans regia*
WATER VIOLET	*Hottonia palustris*
WHITE CHESTNUT	*AEsculus hippocastanum*
WILD OAT	*Bromus ramosus*†
WILD ROSE	*Rosa canina*
WILLOW	*Salix vitellina*

† There is no English name for Bromus ramosus. Bromus is an ancient word meaning Oat. (The alteration in the Latin names of certain of the plants in this edition of *The Twelve Healers* is due to changes of nomenclature governed by The International Rules of Botanical Nomenclature.)

THE COMPOSITE RESCUE REMEDY

Dr. Bach combined five specific Remedies from the 38 to formulate an emergency composite that he chose to call "Rescue Remedy". He saved a fisherman's life in 1930 with this preparation.

Its purpose is to treat the pre or post emotional effect that a sufferer may experience through shock, great fear or terror, panic, severe mental stress and tension, a feeling of desperation or a numbed, bemused state of mind.

To nullify the sufferer's shock and fear is of the utmost importance in helping the natural healing process of one's being to proceed without hindrance. Shock, terror and panic can manifest in minor traumas as well as in the more serious states of emergency. A brief definition of 'emergency' would be e.g. when in mental or physical shock, terror and panic, various emotional upsets (bereavement, stage fright, visiting the dentist, general nervous debility, trauma etc.). Even severe bites and stings create the effects of shock and panic.

Rescue Remedy can be taken along with any of the other 38 Remedies if required – please see general instructions, also for reference to the **RESCUE REMEDY CREAM** preparation.

Note: It has to be remembered that each of the 5

remedies used in this composite can be equally efficient when taken as a separate entity as and when required.

TREATMENT OF ANIMALS

One can sometimes assess a particular personality trait or definite temperamental attitude in animals (viz. aggressiveness, possessiveness, lethargy, timidity, jealous etc.) and so they, as with humans, can be treated accordingly with one or more of the 38 remedies. The Rescue Remedy, although not being considered a panacea for all ills as far as humans are concerned, does act as an excellent all purpose basic remedy for animals, who react very favourably to this remedy irrespective of the state or cause of suffering.

Dosage: 4 drops of the Rescue Remedy stock concentrate (plus 2 drops from any other chosen remedy) in the animal's drink. A dilution can also be sprinkled over its food. For larger creatures needing to drink out of a bucket, the dosage would be in proportion to approximately 10 drops per gallon. 4 drops on a cube of sugar might be appropriate with some animals.

METHODS OF DOSAGE

The stock concentrates issued by the Centre will keep indefinitely. They can be taken by people of all ages – there is no danger of an over-dose or side effects, and should the wrong choice be made no harm will ensue. They will not be influenced by, nor will they effect any form of medicine prescribed to a person.

Animals and plants also benefit from this treatment.

First determine the personality and temperament; fears, worries, emotional upsets and the subsequent effect in outlook and attitude. More than one remedy can be taken at the one time, but it should not be difficult to limit your choice to within six.

DOSAGE: Take 2 drops from each chosen stock remedy in a cup of water, fruit juice, or any beverage, and sip fairly frequently. Replenish cup to continue treatment if need be ... ALTERNATIVELY you can put the drops in a bottle of approx. 1 fl.oz. (30ml) capacity and fill up with Natural Spring Water (non-gas) and take 4 drops on the tongue directly from the bottle. Take as often as needed but at least 4 times a day, especially first and last thing daily.

Hold the dose a moment or so in the mouth before swallowing to gain the full effect (this also applies when sipped from a cup). Such a-prepared dosage bottle will remain fresh for about 3 weeks if stored in a cool place ('fridge in very warm climates), but should a preservative be necessary, include a spoonful of brandy or cider vinegar to the preparation. Dosage drops can be added to a baby's bottle or taken in a spoonful of water.

Rescue Remedy can be included along with the others when needed, but use 4 drops instead of two as indicated for other remedies, and also count it as a single stock remedy rather than the five from which it is composed. When required for immediate or emergency use as a separate remedy take 4 drops in a cup of water and sip at intervals. If the sufferer is unable to swallow, or in a comatose state, then the lips, behind the ears and the wrists should be moistened with the Remedy. **It does not take the place of medical attention.**

External Application. For burns, scalds, stings, sprains etc. - apply a couple of drops direct from the Rescue Remedy stock bottle immediately to the effected area

There is also available **Rescue Remedy Cream** (non lanolin, Homoeopathically prepared base) for ulcers, lacerations, burns, scalds, sprains, massage and many other needs.

Note: If liquid is totally unavailable, then drops *can* be taken from the stock concentrate, but it must be emphasised for the benefit of abstainers, that this would mean a direct intake of brandy.

And may we ever have joy and gratitude in our hearts that the Great Creator of all things, in His Love for us, has placed the herbs in the fields for our healing.

www.ingramcontent.com/pod-product-compliance
Lightning Source LLC
Chambersburg PA
CBHW021917160426
42813CB00097B/272